Fake Hair, Don't Care

How to Choose the Best Hair Extension Method to Protect and Grow Your Natural Hair

By B. CliShea

Fake Hair, Don't Care. How to Choose the Best Hair Extension Method to Protect and Grow Your Natural Hair

By B. CliShea

First Edition

https://www.clishea.co

Cover & Interior layout design by Mariana Vidakovics De Victor

Images from: https://pixabay.com/

Disclaimer
The information provided within this book is for general informational purposes only. While we try to keep the information up-to-date and correct, there are no representations or warranties, express or implied, about the completeness, accuracy, reliability, suitability or availability with respect to the information, products, services, or related graphics contained in this book for any purpose. Any use of this information is at your own risk.

The methods described within this book are the author's personal thoughts. They are not intended to be a definitive set of instructions for this project. You may discover there are other methods and materials to accomplish the same end result.

CONTENTS

Introduction

Your hair is constantly exposed to damaging elements such as wind, dry air, sand, pollution and UV rays. And you know what makes it worse? When you do decide to style your hair, you could end up with even more damage. One reason is that many hair products these days are too harsh. In addition, styling hair usually requires applying heat, causing it to become frizzy and brittle. The good news is, there IS a way for you to have stunning hairstyle AND keep your hair healthy – hair extensions.

Hair extensions can give that much-needed cover while giving you the look and style you want. They can help you protect your scalp and roots, which also helps promote healthier hair growth. Hair extensions can also complement a wide range of hairstyles.

You have short hair but you want to try having long, flowing hair? Hair extensions can let you do so. You have a no-nonsense shoulder-length hairstyle but you want to have dramatic long curls for a gala? Get some hair extensions and in a matter of hours, you can sport voluminous, smooth, curly locks. If you're facing hair loss, hair extensions can also help by covering bald spots.

These hair extensions come in various shade, styles, materials, textures and lengths. Most of these can be styled just like your own natural hair. These can be installed to your hair seamlessly and no one will know you are even wearing any. For example, a few well-placed curled hair extension clip-ins can be handy if you want to look extra sexy on a date.

Hair extensions aren't just for giving you a whole new look or covering bald spots. Even if you already have nice-looking hair, they can make your hairstyle look even more fabulous. Yes, hair extensions allow you to change your look without putting your hair through various potentially damaging hair styling processes. In fact, this book is not just about hair extension styles in general but will also cover one important purpose of hair extensions- hair protection and growth.

If you want to protect your hair from

damaging elements but wish to still look stylish, you can use hair extensions to protect your scalp as new hair grows.

The head is covered with hair extensions so that the real hair underneath does not get exposed to harmful chemicals and environmental stress. This protection can help the roots to grow out new, healthier hair.

This book will show you the many hair extension methods you can try. You will also learn important information about each of the methods such as how long it will take to install, how much maintenance is needed and so on.

This book will also show you how to properly take care of the hair extensions you wish to use. That includes care before installation, while wearing the extensions, right before removal and most importantly, after the extensions are removed.

Read on and find out how you can improve your locks with some pretty hair extensions.

To thank you for your purchase,
you're entitled to a special giveaway.[1]

---

[1] https://www.instafreebie.com/free/xNCiP

Types of Hair Extension Methods

There are different kinds of hair extensions. Before you go to the salon and get hair extensions, take some time to understand these lovely add-ons. Know the different types available, the cost and most especially, the amount of maintenance needed.

Hair Extension Method #1
Tape-in Extensions

Description:

This is the newest extension method currently available. The extensions are applied to the natural hair through either a single-sided or a double-sided polyurethane tape.

Double-sided tape is more often used for general hair conditions. This can be used on all types of hair, from thin hair to thick and curly locks.

The backing is removed from the weft before it is applied. The weft is attached to the hair. Another weft is then attached to the tape's other side. This will be sandwiching the natural hair between two wefts.

The downside is that the weight of the 2 wefts may pull on thin natural hair. This can causer hair breakage off or pull hair out from its roots. An alternative is to use single-sided tape connection.

Single-sided tape is more often used on those who have extremely thin or brittle natural hair. This attachment is also recommended for thin hair over the side of the head and around the temples.

The weft applied is as a single panel. The natural hair will not be sandwiched between 2 wefts. This will be lighter on the roots yet still give a nice natural look to your overall hairstyle.

Installation Duration:

This takes the least time in applying compared to other strand-by-strand hair extensions. The volume applications usually take around 20 to 30 minutes only. Full applications usually take around 45 to 60 minutes.

Cost (US Standards):

$ to $$$$

The cost mainly depends on the brand of the wefts used and how many panels or boxes of hair will be used. The type of hair will also affect how much this hair extension type will cost. The fee for application also varies.

The price range is usually around $200 to $800.

Maintenance:

Hair can be styled as normal. Just remember never to use any products that contain oil or silicon on the roots of natural hair and on the adhesive. Brush hair daily, starting from the root of the natural hair to the tip of the hair extension.

Hair Extension Method #2
GLUE-IN

DESCRIPTION:

As the name implies, glue is used to attach the weft to the natural hair. Glue is placed on the base of the weft before it is attached. The wefts last for only a few days. The wefts can be removed from the hair by applying an oil-based solvent.

INSTALLATION DURATION:

Temporary. The wefts will have to be removed and reapplied every few days or after taking a shower.

COST (US STANDARDS):

$ to $$; least expensive of all types of hair extensions

The wefts have to be reapplied after a shower or every few days.

Hair Extension Method #3
BRAIDED OR SEW-IN FULL WEAVE

DESCRIPTION:

This type of hair extension is more widely known as the weave. This is the ideal type for those who have thick, coarse, or curly hair. Thin, weak, damaged or fine hair may not be able to hold the weight of a weave, especially a full weave. However, the stylist may be able to make a few tweaks to properly install a weave despite these hair conditions.

A base is needed to serve as attachment of the extensions. The base is created by braiding the natural hair tightly against the scalp. The wefts are attached to the hair by sewing them into the braid with a needle and thread.

Installation Duration:

How long it takes the weave to be installed depends on the amount to be installed. A partial head of weave can take a few hours to be installed. A full head will take much longer.

The lifespan of the weave depends not only on the quality of the hair extensions. How well your own natural hair can hold up to the tension of the braids and the pull of the hair extension weight is also a factor. In general, weaves should be removed after 6 to 8 weeks. Some can last for about 2 to 3 months.

Always have the tracks and the braids checked. New hair can grow over the braids and the tracks. Leaving the weave longer will cause the new hair growth to become tangled and matted.

Cost (US Standards):

$ to $$

This is among the most expensive hair extensions, mainly because of the amount of work it requires for proper application. Cost of the hair depends on the quality, length, volume and styling requirements.

The usual price ranges around $400 to up to more than $2000.

Maintenance:

Hair must be washed regularly. Styling the weave comes with very limited options. Overstyling may cause the braids to become loose. The weave, though, can be straightened, curled and/or shampooed in the same way as normal hair.

Hair Extension Method #4
Keratin Bond

Description:

This type is also known as pre-bonded or glue-in hair extension. This type attaches a weft to your natural hair using adhesives.

There are many subtypes of keratin bond hair extensions. There is the keratin U-tip, hard bond and soft bond. This type also includes the glue-in hair extension.

Keratin U-tip

The keratin U-tip is a type of hair extension technique where the extension is attached to normal hair strand by strand. The bonds are lined with silicon then attached to hair with the application of a heating element.

The normal hair is neatly arranged in between the U-tip. A hot extension tool is placed between the connections to melt the bond. This attaches the hair extension to normal hair.

These bonds are applied very near the root of the normal hair. This makes it look like the extension is real hair connected to the scalp via the hair root. This creates a more natural look to the hair, with movements that look very natural as well.

Hard Bond

This type uses glue to attach the hair extension to sections of your hair. These are rigid and oftentimes uncomfortable. The hair does not freely move like your natural hair does. This type usually lasts for only about 4 to 6 weeks. It has to be maintained frequently by a professional stylist.

Using this type of bond comes with a high risk of damaging your natural hair. This is also usually more expensive because of the price of the hair used for the extension and the effort it takes for application.

Soft Bond

This is more comfortable to use than the hard bond type. The attachment is also more flexible, which allows for greater hair movement. The adhesive used is made from acrylic-based or latex-based materials.

Installation Duration:

This method takes quite some time to apply, with the duration averaging around 6 to 8 hours. Experienced hairdressers typically apply this within 2 to 3 hours.

Keratin bond hair extensions typically last for around 3 months. High quality materials with regular maintenance can make it last for up to 4 to 5 months.

Cost (US Standards):

Price varies, depending on the brand and the amount of strands to be attached. Cost of application is also a factor.

The average cost is around $400 to $2000.

Maintenance:

Avoid over-styling as this will the hair extensions to wear out sooner. Too much heat or styling products can weigh down the hair, including the roots of your own natural hair. Give your hair and your scalp time to relax and breathe without the stress of too much styling and styling products.

Avoid using any oil-based products on the hair extensions. This can damage the bonds and cause your hair extensions to slip out of their attachment.

Cold Fusion

Description:

This method is also called micro link, micro-ring, or micro-bead hair extension.

For this method, small sections of natural hair are pulled through small locks or beads. The beads are then clamped shut using a special tool. Reliable salons use cylinders made of copper and lined with silicon. The lining helps in protecting the natural hair.

Installation Duration:

This type of hair extension is among those that can take quite a longer time for application. It typically takes about 4 to 6 hours. Experienced hair stylists typically attach I-tips in 2 to 3 hours. Some can take around 4 to 6 hours.

The hair extensions typically last for about 3 to 4 months, with regular styling and frequent maintenance.

Cost (US Standards):

Cost depends on the brand and on the amount of strands applied to the client's hair. The price range usually falls within a range of $400 to more than $2000.

Maintenance:

Avoid using silicon-containing and oil-based products over the area where extensions and natural hair are attached to each other.

Hair Extension Method #6
Clip-Ins

Description:

These temporary hair extensions are typically used for special events or occasions. The wefts are attached to a metal clip, which are then attached or clipped into the natural hair. These are typically available in varying lengths, ranging from 2 to 8 inches.

These are removed before bedtime. Otherwise, the wefts will rub against the pillow and form nasty tangles.

Some temporary hair extensions come with undetectable wires instead of large metal clips. These are often more commonly known as halo hair extensions.

Halo extensions

This type comes in a weft attached to a very thin wire. The wire is placed on the head, wearing it like a halo or a crown. A section of your natural hair is pulled through and over the wire to hide from sight and make your hair and the hair extension look like a continuous unit.

INSTALLATION DURATION:

Very temporary - you can put this in or take it out anytime you want. You can do this on your own or have a stylist add it to your hair to match the hair style you want.

For the halo extension, despite the larger volume, it only takes about a minute to place on your head. For clip-ins with smaller sections of hair, it takes a mere few seconds. The same is with removal. It's all easy, convenient and no-fuss.

The lifespan of the hair extensions depends on the quality of material and frequency of use. These can break down quite easily with daily use, including daily wash, wear and styling. How often it gets heat styled is also a factor in how soon the hair extensions wear out.

These extensions can be worn all day but needs to be removed before you go to bed.

Cost (US Standards):

$ to $$

These are most probably the cheapest types of hair extensions but not necessarily of the lowest quality. Price typically falls within the range of $150 to $300.

For the halo extension, the price typically falls within the range $229 to $269.

Clip-in hair extensions should be washed infrequently. If it becomes dull or dry, you can apply some deep conditioner. Comb extensions regularly to keep it tangle-free. A Loop brush or wide-toothed comb should be used.

Hair Extension Method #7
STOCK WIGS

DESCRIPTION:

These are made from synthetic materials. Stock wigs are mass produced, in limited styles. These are also machine-made. The synthetic hair fibers are sewn into wefts then sewn into caps for easier wearing/taking off.

INSTALLATION DURATION:

These are easy to put on, usually taking a few minutes, around 10 to 15 minutes.

These wigs are made of synthetic materials and tend to last for quite a longer time. However, these will not last very long if shampooed and styled too frequently.

Cost (US Standards):

These can go for very cheap to a bit expensive. Price range usually starts from $5 to about a couple hundred.

Maintenance:

This type requires little maintenance. It can even be worn straight out of the box.

Hair Extension Method #8
Semi-custom-made Wigs

Description:

These are made with a combination of natural hairs and synthetic hair fibers. These are partially made by a machine then finished off by hand. The top portion is a solid wefted cap. The sides are of fine mesh netting.

Installation Duration:

These are easy to put on and take off. It may take a few minutes to about an hour depending on the style desired.

The strands typically last for about 4 to 6 months, with proper maintenance.

Cost (US Standards):

Price range typically less than $100 up to about $1000, depending on amount of human hair and quality of construction.

Maintenance:

This type requires regular washing and styling to keep the strands tangle-free and looking good.

Hair Extension Method #9
CUSTOM-MADE WIGS

DESCRIPTION:

These are made with a combination of natural hair strands and synthetic hair fibers. The strands are hand tied on a stretchy piece of fine mesh netting. This is called custom-made because it is manufactured according to the exact measurements of the client.

INSTALLATION DURATION:

The strands can last for up to a year or more, if maintained properly.

COST (US STANDARDS):

The cost depends on how much natural human hair was used on the wigs and the length and style. It can easily range from around a few hundred dollars to a little more than a $1000.

Maintenance:

This type requires some careful styling and regular maintenance. It has to be washed frequently to free the human hair strand components clear of dirt and oil.

Hair Extension Method #10
Crochet Braids

Description:

This is actually a term used on how extensions are added to the hair. Instead of sewing in, taping, bonding, taping or gluing, the hair wefts are crocheted into your hair. Your natural hair is braided or made into cornrows. The extensions are then attached one-by-one by crocheting it into the braids or cornrows.

Installation Duration:

Crochet braids are installed within 3 hours. This may vary depending on the amount of packs to be installed and the style.

The packs can last usually for about 4 to 8 weeks.

Cost (US Standards):

Price range depends on the number of packs to be used on the hair. Usually, it tales around 4 to 7 packs. Each pack usually costs around $3 to $10.

Maintenance:

Maintenance is minimal and does not have to be washed regularly.

Hair Extension Method #11
Extensions braided with natural hair

Description:

This is one of the oldest types of hair extensions. The hair is braided then braided extensions are braided in as well.

Installation Duration:

This method can last for a few hours, around 3 to 4 hours depending on amount of hair to braid, length, style and amount of braid extensions.

This can be allowed to stay on the hair for 2 months. Remove after 2 months or else lose more hair to tangle, knots and increased hair shedding.

Cost (US Standards):

This type of hair extension typically costs around $50 to about $300 or so.

Maintenance:

The scalp is pretty much exposed in this type of hair extension. Apply gentle shampoo on the scalp and rub gently with your fingertips or a soft cloth. Rinse under running water and allow the water to bring the shampoo flowing through the hair inside the braids. This type also needs regular moisturizing.

Summary of Hair Extension Methods

<table>
<tr><td colspan="2" align="center">Skin/ Tape Weft</td></tr>
<tr>
<td rowspan="4">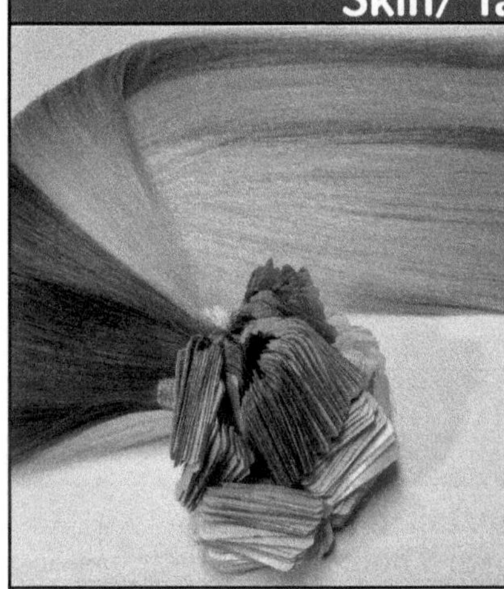</td>
<td>Installation Duration
• Volume applications around 20 to 30 minutes
• Full applications around 45 to 60 minutes</td>
</tr>
<tr><td>Durability
• About 5 to 6 months</td></tr>
<tr><td>Cost
• $200 to $800</td></tr>
<tr><td>Maintenance
• can be styled as normal</td></tr>
<tr><td colspan="2" align="center">Glue Bond</td></tr>
<tr>
<td rowspan="4">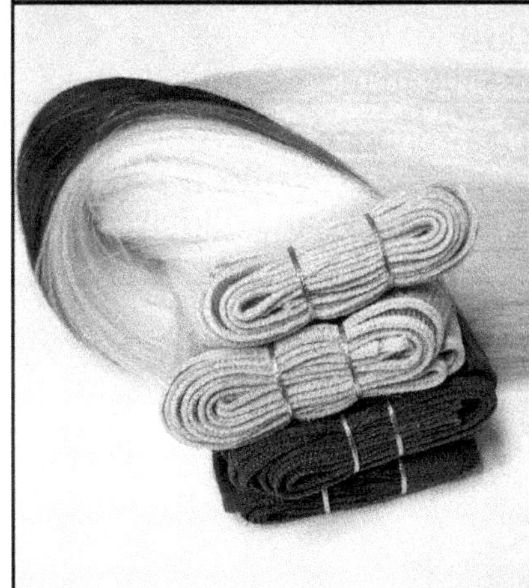</td>
<td>Installation Duration
• removed and reapplied every few days or after taking a shower</td>
</tr>
<tr><td>Durability
• 3 months</td></tr>
<tr><td>Cost
• $400 to more than $2000</td></tr>
<tr><td>Maintenance
• wefts have to be reapplied after a shower or every few days</td></tr>
</table>

Sew-In Full Weave

	Installation Duration • About 2 to 3 hours by a professional
	Durability • 2 to 3 months
	Cost • $400 to more than $2000
	Maintenance • washed regularly with minimal styling options

Fusion

Keratin/ Hot fusion	Cold fusion (Microbeads/ Microlinks/Brazilian knot)
Installation Duration • apply this within 2 to 3 hours	**Installation Duration** • to 6 hours
Durability • around 3 to 5 months	**Durability** • 3 to 4 months
Cost • $400 to $2000	**Cost** • $400 to more than $2000
Maintenance • avoid too much heat, products and styling	**Maintenance** • Avoid use of silicon-containing and oil-based products

Clip-ins

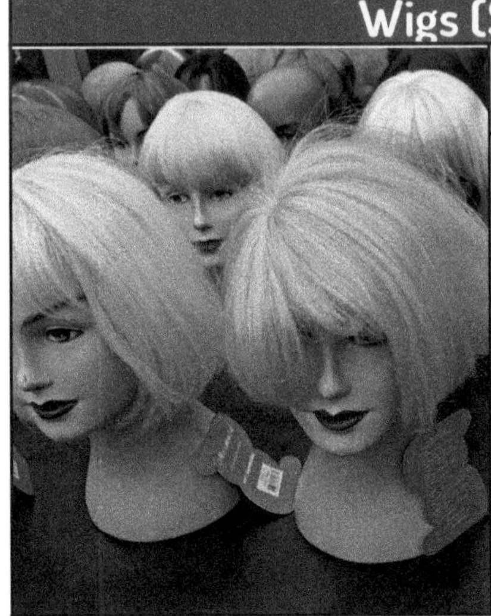

Installation Duration
•10 minutes

Durability
•depends on the quality of material and frequency of use

Cost
•$150 to $300

Maintenance
•washed infrequently

Wigs (Stock)

Installation Duration
•around 10 to 15 minutes

Durability
•last for quite a longer time, depending on quality of material and frequency of use

Cost
•$5 to about a couple hundred

Maintenance
•Minimal maintenance

Wigs (Semi-custom)

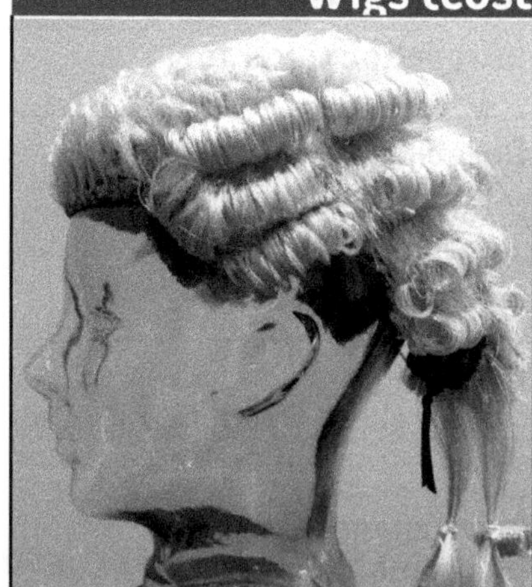

Installation Duration	• around 10 to 15 minutes, to an hour
Durability	• about 4 to 6 months
Cost	• less than $100 up to about $1000
Maintenance	• regular washing and styling

Wigs (custom-made)

Installation Duration	• around 10 to 15 minutes, to an hour
Durability	• up to a year or more
Cost	• few hundred dollars to a little more than a $1000
Maintenance	• some careful styling and regular maintenance

Crochet braids

Installation Duration
- 3 hours

Durability
- 4 to 8 weeks

Cost
- $3 to $10 per pack

Maintenance
- does not have to be washed regularly

Extensions braided with natural hair

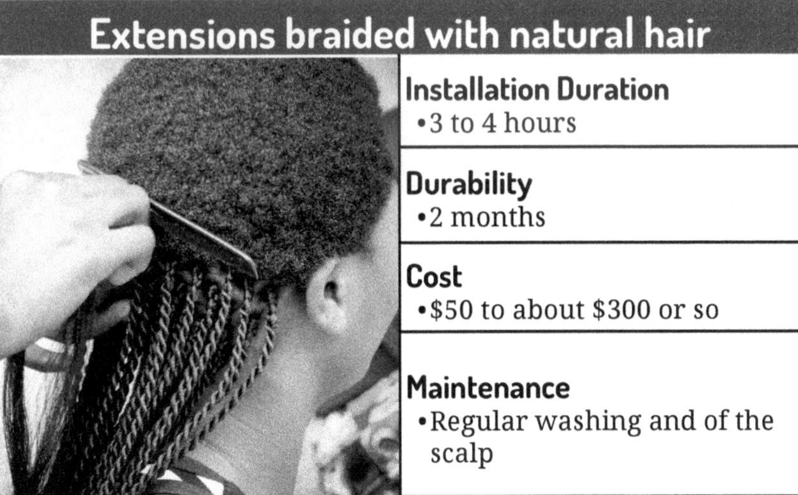

Installation Duration
- 3 to 4 hours

Durability
- 2 months

Cost
- $50 to about $300 or so

Maintenance
- Regular washing and of the scalp

Which Hair Extension Method Protects & Grows Your Hair the Best?

Hair extensions work differently for different people. Some people experience greater hair protection and hair regrowth with weaves while some are better off with halo extensions.

This is a general guide to the level of protection certain types of hair extensions provide. This guide is based on how much the extension method can keep hair from damage and how much it can help promote healthy hair growth.

HAIR PROTECTION RATING SCALE EXPLAINED

In this section, we will examine the general hair protection rating capability of each of the discussed hair extension types in the previous section. This section uses three categories to rate the protection capabilities. These are:

*Limited protection = means that only a small area can be protected from exposure to factors that can cause hair loss and weaken/damage the hair

*Moderate Protection = means that hair is well protected but protection is mostly limited to the area covered by the amount and volume of the weft. This also means that the protective abilities of the hair extension method depend on how well the extension is applied. Poor application creates more damage than provide protection.

*Complete Protection = means that your entire head is protected against damaging factors to your hair.

» Tape/Skin Weft

Suitable for:

All types of hair, usually for those with thin to medium density

The tapes do not cause much damage on the hair strands. Tape-ins are also lightweight that it does not promote hair loss or balding. Your own hair remains intact as it grows protected from the damaging effects of UV, environmental pollutants and similar substances.

If you are looking for hair extension for style and looks alone, then tape-ins are a great choice. These are least likely to pull your hair or give undue strain on your scalp.

If you are looking for something to complement the hair you are trying to grow out, this is also a good choice. It is lightweight and can grow out along with your natural hair.

Protection rating:

Moderate to complete protection

Moderate because this depends on the amount of wefts used and how well the tapes are applied. Poorly applied tapes may damage the ends of your natural hair.

» Glue

Suitable for: Any hair type

Protection rating: Moderate

In terms of covering the hair against damaging elements, glue-in hair extensions can work. However, the glue itself may be irritating to the scalp. It may damage sensitive hair and cause some hair growth problems instead of promoting a full head of healthy, strong new hair.

» Keratin Bond

Suitable for:

Hair with medium to thick density

Protection rating: moderate

This can help protect the hair from damage as it grows. One downside is that the heat application during installation may cause damage enough to cause hair loss or weak hair growth.

» Sew-in Weave (full)

Suitable for: any hair type

Protection rating: complete

This can cover your head and protect your hair from harmful heat styling, exposure to environmental pollutants and to some extent, from harmful UV rays. Your hair is essentially covered and allowed to recover and regrow. However, this highly depends if the weave is applied properly.

» Sew-in Weave (partial)

Suitable for: any hair type

Protection rating: moderate

The limited area covered by the weave also limits its protective capability. However, this is still a good choice in protecting your hair as it regrows.

» Cold Fusion – Brazilian Knot

Suitable for: all hair types

Protection rating: complete

These are lightweight and non-irritating on the hair strands, the roots and even at the attachment points.

» Cold Fusion – Micolink/microbead

Suitable for:

Hair with medium to thick density

Protection rating: moderate

Protection is moderate, as long as it is applied properly. If not, greater tension will exist and it will pull on your scalp and hair roots. This can worsen hair loss. New hair growth will be thin and weak because of the stress present while the hair is growing.

This hair extension method should not be attached too close to the scalp. This can impede normal hair growth as well as pull on the scalp too much. These should be clipped to just the right amount of natural hair. Otherwise, the weft may be too heavy for a thin bundle of natural of hair. The weight may not be properly supported, leading to breakage of your natural hair.

» Clip-in/Clip-on

Suitable for: medium density

Protection rating: Low

Some clip-ins hair extensions are heavy and pull on your hair roots. The weight of the m metal clips alone can weaken your hair roots and promote hair loss.

Heavy daily usage is also discouraged, especially when the sets weigh more than 180 grams. This can give considerable amount of strain on your scalp and natural hair.

» Crochet Braids

Protection rating: low

The protection is limited to the coverage. It does coverage a large area. However, the braid used can be damaging. The braid pattern commonly used as base for crochet braids can damage the edges. This tends to promote receding hairline. The cornrows used as alternative can sometimes lead to hair breakage.

» Wig

Suitable for: all hair types

Protection rating: moderate to complete

The entire head is covered by the wig and protected from damaging elements. However, check the quality of the cap. It should be breathable material. Otherwise, you scalp won't be able to breathe. It will quickly become hot and will essentially "cook" your hair roots. This goes whether you will be wearing to wig for a few hours or for an entire day.

ADDITIONAL GUIDELINES

The number one thing to consider is the condition of your hair. Is it strong? Is it thick? Is it fine and thin? That will determine the weight and volume of the hair extensions that you can apply to your head. Despite a high protection rating for a certain hair extension type, you won't be able to optimize its benefits if it isn't suited for your hair type.

In general, you would not want to install a very heavy weave if your hair is fine and brittle. Weave typically provides moderate to complete protection against hair damage from exposure to elements. However, it may produce greater damage because of the weight, which fine and thin hair may not be able to support. So instead of protecting your locks, you might be damaging them.

On the other hand, a lightweight weft hair extension can give you the complete protection you need despite a low protection rating on this scale. For instance, you do have good overall hair health condition but your roots are weak. Hair is fine and thin, although shiny, smooth and otherwise healthy. A lightweight tape-in is a good quality wig can be a better choice.

Should You Use Synthetic Or Human Hair?

One of the biggest questions to face is whether to choose extensions or wigs made with real human hair or one with synthetic fibers. The answer depends on a lot of factors. Each choice comes with pros and cons.

Human hair extensions/wigs were made using real hair. The hair strands come from salons. There are some places where a person can go and sell his/her hair. The harvested human hair is cleaned, styled and made into various types of hair extensions. These are, of course, more natural looking and feel more natural when worn. The feel and the texture is the same as the natural hair. It can be washed and styled in the same manner, too.

Synthetic wigs and extension are created to look like natural human hair. High quality ones also feel and move just like natural human hair.

Hair Extensions Made with Human Hair

Pros

Styling versatility

Since the wig or hair extension is made from real human hair, it can be styled practically in the same manner as the hair growing on your scalp. It can be colored, styled, even permed. However, there are certain precautions that need to be done when styling hair extensions made from human hair. These may be the same as the hair on your scalp but it is no longer being nourished by your scalp. It has to be given some extra care to keep the hair extension look healthy and last longer. Styling is most recommended to be left to stylists with experience working with human hair wigs or extensions.

Texture

Human hair extensions or wigs come in different textures, just like real hair growing from the scalp. You can choose from various textures, such as thin and fine, coarse and thick, etc. Clients can choose the hair extension that closely matches the texture of their own hair. This will help the hair extension to blend better with the wearer's real hair.

Longevity

Hair extensions made with human hair tend to last long with proper maintenance. Some high quality brands can last for about a year or more even with daily use.

Look

Extensions made with human hair look more natural and blends well with the wearer's own natural hair.

Cons

High maintenance

Your own hair growing from your scalp is being nourished by the blood that flows through your scalp. The scalp also produces oils that serve to moisturize and keep your hair healthy. Hair extensions using human hair do not get nourished in this same manner. Hence, it has to be maintained more regularly.

Human hair extensions need to be washed frequently and deeply conditioned. It also has to be styled regularly to keep it looking good and feel more natural.

Cost

These hair extensions tend to be more expensive because of all the careful processes needed to keep the harvested human hair looking great, natural and healthy.

Color variations

It is difficult to find the same exact shade of one batch of human hair extensions. Buying a new one may not be of the same exact shade as the previous one. This is because hair used for these extensions came from multiple sources. One way to get around this is to have the hair extension colored to your desired shade before using.

Color fading

Hair extensions made with real human hair can be colored and turn out in the same way as when coloring real hair growing on your head. However, the color can change as it oxidizes. The color may also fade as it is repeatedly exposed to light.

Weather response

Just like your own hair, human hair extensions would also react to weather. It can get frizzy with humidity, become dry in hot weather or turn limp.

Fragile

The extensions will be prone to damage, breakage and faster wearing out with overstyling. Too frequent use of heated styling tools can destroy the strands. Back-combing and harsh brushing may also damage the hair strands, just like it would on your natural hair.

Heavier

Human hair wigs and hair extensions tend to be heavier compared to synthetic ones of the same length, volume and style. This is worth considering if using a large volume and for an extended period. The heaviness can pull on your natural hair strands. This can put you at higher risk for traction or tension alopecia. This can also make it more uncomfortable to use over extended periods, depending on the type of extension you wear, i.e., weaves.

Styling

It will usually take more skill and effort to style hair extensions made with human hair. It is more recommended to leave the styling to experts. It is also more labor intensive.

Synthetic hair extensions

Pros

Easy to maintain

The synthetic fibers do not get damaged easily in the same manner as human hair does. This makes hair extensions made with synthetic fibers easier to take care of.

These extensions usually come with "style retention". These mean that these hair extensions do not have to be styled. Wash the hair as usual, shake and allow to dry. It will return naturally into the initial style without any further effort from you.

Style memory

In the same way, synthetic hair extensions retain their style regardless of what weather they get exposed in.

Versatility

You can buy various hair extensions in

different styles and colors to use. Just change the extension when you want to change the color and the style. You do not have to go to a stylist for this.

However, this is applicable for temporary hair extension types. It will be difficult to change synthetic hair extensions such as weaves and glue-ins on your own whenever you feel like changing your look.

Color selection

Synthetic hair extensions come in a large selection of colors. Choices range from natural hair colors to various shades of fantasy colors such as bubblegum pink and neon green.

Cost

Most synthetic hair extensions are inexpensive. However, some top quality ones that look, feel, move and styled like normal human hair can be quite expensive, too.

Low maintenance

Synthetic hair fibers do not need much care.

It does not have to be washed and conditioned as often as natural hair.

Cons

Unnatural shine

Some cheap, low quality synthetic hair extensions may have an unnatural shine to it.

Longevity

Most synthetic hair extensions do not last very long like ones made with real human hair. Most typically lasts for only 4 to 6 months when worn daily.

Less versatility

Most synthetic hair extensions do not do well when a heated tool is applied to it. These usually cannot be curled or straightened. However, some brands offer "heat-friendly" synthetic hair extensions that can be styled safely with heated tools like curling irons and hair straighteners.

No changing colors

Changing hair colors with synthetic hair extensions mean changing the entire extension. You can't have synthetic hair colored in the same way as normal natural hair. Most traditional hair colors do not stick to the synthetic hair fibers.

"HEAT-FRIENDLY" SYNTHETIC HAIR EXTENSIONS

Pros

Style versatility

These hair extensions can be styled and restyled in any way, even with the use of heated styling equipment.

Style retention

Even the heat-friendly synthetic hair extensions come with this same feature as the traditional synthetic ones. Wash the hair extension, allow to air dry and it will go back to the style it was originally made into. For instance, you bought hair extensions in large voluminous waves. After washing and air-drying, the hair extension will return to its wavy style. You do not have to style the extension into this heat-styled look anymore.

More natural look

This type of synthetic hair extension usually is less shiny compared to traditional ones. This reduced shine makes it look a little bit more natural, like real human hair.

Consistency

These usually look and feel a bit more like real human hair but do not react to weather. It does not get frizzy, limp or dry depending on the type of weather.

Cost-effective

Some of the top quality heat-friendly synthetic wigs look so much like real human hair. They also feel and move in the same way as real hair. They can also be styled in the same but without the high maintenance needs of human hair extensions.

This type may be as expensive as top quality human hair extension. However, it can turn out to be more cost-effective eventually because of all the other advantages. Examples will be les maintenance needs, style retention (for less effort on styling) and texture consistency.

Cons

Texture

Even if these are heat-friendly, the synthetic fibers may still get damaged. Small, tight curls may form and make it difficult to tame and style the hair extension. These can form when the hair extension is excessively restyled. Abrasion or getting the strands rubbed against surfaces such as the back of the seat or a pillow may also cause texture problems.

Longevity

Heat-friendly synthetic hair extensions only

last for a few months. This type wears out sooner than hair extensions made with real hair or synthetic fibers.

Coloring

These hair extensions cannot be colored in the same way as real human hair. Colors do not stick to the synthetic fibers that well.

Require advanced styling skills

This type of hair extension can be restyled but it will require some advanced skills. Styling heat-friendly hair extensions is a bit more difficult than when working with human hair. This can be quite a challenge for most.

FACTORS TO CONSIDER IN CHOOSING BETWEEN SYNTHETIC AND HUMAN HAIR

Aside from understanding the pros and cons of each hair type, it is also important to consider a few other factors.

Budget

As previously mentioned, hair extensions that use human hair are more expensive than synthetic ones. Top quality ones can reach well over a few hundred dollars compared to about less than $100 for most synthetic hair extensions.

Because synthetic hair extensions are cheap, they may be a better a choice if the hair extension is meant for temporary or short-term use only. This type may also be worn for longer periods but there would be the added cost of maintenance. Good quality ones that can last longer may also be a bit pricier.

If use is daily and expected to last for more than a few months, it may be better to spend a little more for hair extensions made with real hair.

Where You'll Be Using Them

Think of the places you will be wearing the hair extensions. Weather will affect the look, feel, texture and movement of the hair extensions, just like your own real hair.

If you are in a humid and hot place or if it gets very damp most of the time, it is recommended to use synthetic hair extensions. These do not get affected by the weather conditions. The style remains the same without taking any extra precautions.

If you prefer to use extensions made with human hair in these types of weather, it is better to get one with shorter and more manageable hair strands. This will be easier to manage and style.

Remember that the quality of the hair extensions, whether synthetic or real human hair, will degrade when exposed outdoors. Direct sunlight can fade the colors. It can also make the hair extension wear out faster.

Frequency of use

Daily use can wear out the hair extensions faster. Those made with real human hair can last up to a year or so with daily use. Synthetic hair extensions would usually last between 4 and 6 months of daily use. Heat-friendly extensions can only last up to 3 months of daily use.

The frequency of use will determine the amount of washing. Frequent use means frequent washing (and styling) and faster wearing out.

How To Properly Remove Hair Extensions

No matter how great your hair extensions are, they will have to be removed eventually. These are not meant to be permanently worn. Some type of hair extensions will have to be removed by an expert stylist at the salon, such as a weave. Some types you can remove by yourself at home. Proper removal and after-care treatment of your real hair are very important to protect your newly grown hair.

» Removing bonded hair extensions

1. Ponytail

Put all hair into a high ponytail. This will help you work systematically in removing the hair extensions. Some bonds may be more obvious than others so work meticulously.

2. Start at the nape of the neck

Untie a small section of your hair at the base of your head, near the nape. Insert a salon comb (the thin end) into the lower portion of the pony tail. You may also use your fingers. Insert then pull out a small section of your hair.

3. Break the bonds

Use a pair of pliers to crimp the bonds. Loosen and then break bonds one at a time. A pair of needle-nose pliers can work more efficiently. Squeeze the bond until it breaks.

When you hear or feel the bond crack, move the pliers to another portion of the bond. Squeeze the pliers again to crack another section of the bond. This will make it much easier to remove the bond later.

4. Oil the bonds

Dip your fingers into an oil mixture. Recommendations include mixture of oils good for the hair such as almond oil, coconut, olive or baby oil.

Rub a small amount of oil over the cracks on the bond. Leave the oil on the bond for 10 to 15 minutes. This will allow the oil time enough to break the keratin and loosen the connection between your real hair and the hair extension.

You may also use a special product designed to dissolve the keratin bond. Alcohol-based gel or acetone may also be applied on the bond. This is effective in dissolving the keratin quickly. Use only a tiny amount to avoid irritating the scalp.

Once the keratin bond is dissolved, you can gently pull out the hair extension. You may even use a comb, running it through the connection and dislodge the hair extension.

5. Apply heat

You can apply heat to the bonds to speed up the breakdown. Set a blow-dryer on low and direct the hot air over the bonds. Apply heat for about 5 to 15 minutes. This will make it easier to slide the hair off from the bond.

6. Pull the bond away from the hair.

Hold your natural hair by the roots to prevent it from getting pulled out too. Hold the roots with one hand and pull the bond out lightly with the other hand.

If you feel the roots are being tugged, stop pulling the bond off. Get the pliers and re-crack the bonds. Apply more oil and wait for a few more minutes before trying to pull the bonds away again.

7. Comb the hair.

Comb the hair with combination brushes to remove any debris or stray hair extensions. First, run a wide-toothed comb through the section of the hair you are currently working on. Next, run a fine-toothed comb. The wide-toothed comb can also gently remove any tangles before the fine-toothed comb passes through.

8. Clean and treat.

Wash your natural hair with clarifying shampoo after all the bonds are removed. This will remove all remaining glue as well as clear away the oils you applied on your hair.

Apply conditioner after rinsing the clarifying shampoo. This will restore nutrients that might have been stripped away by the products you applied to remove the bonds.

How To Care For Your Hair After Removing Extensions

After-care starts before the hair extensions were even removed. Regularly check or have an expert check your natural hair. You should never forget to take care of your natural hair as you let it grow underneath your hair extensions.

Washing, cleansing and conditioning schedule depends on the type of hair extension you have. Whenever you clean your hair, make sure to clean up to the roots of your natural hair. Dirt, oil, wax and residue from the products you apply to your hair and hair extensions can build up on your scalp. This can clog your hair follicles and hinder normal hair growth.

Cleanse well especially around the root area. Use sulfate-free shampoo and massage it well on your scalp. Rinse well too. Residue from the shampoo, even if it is the mildest one, can still cause a few problems later on.

You may also use herbal calming spray products on your scalp. This can help relieve the tension on the roots from the weight of the hair extensions.

» Check for hair shedding vs hair loss

After the extensions are removed, a few strands of hair are expected to fall off. It is normal to find quite a number of strands shed on a daily basis.

The amount of shedding depends on the type of hair extensions you had installed. If you wore more hair extensions or heavier ones, expect to have a bit more hair shedding compared to when you use few strands of extensions with lighter bonds.

Hair shedding is not hair loss. Shedding is a normal occurrence. We shed hair daily. It's the old or weak hairs that we shed to make way for new hair growths.

After the removal of the hair extensions, there may be a larger amount of hair shedding. This is from the buildup of hair stored within the braids.

» Be gentle

Hair extensions apply some amount of strain on your hair roots, especially if worn for an extended period. Once off, your hair will be very sensitive. The slightest tug will be uncomfortable and may even lead to damage.

This is why it is better to get the extensions removed by a professional. The professional hair stylist can immediately provide the care your hair needs, depending on how it will appear. For example, after removal, your natural hair looks thin, fine and frizzy. The professional hairstylist will be able to handle the removal more carefully then apply the professional product gentle enough to solve the problem.

»Let the scalp breathe

Even with the most meticulous regular washing and treatment, a small amount of buildup will still form underneath the hair extensions and the braid.

Cleanse the scalp gently right after the removal of the extensions. Remove all the buildup to allow the scalp to breathe and restore to good health.

Deep cleanse with a gentle yet powerful dandruff shampoo to really dislodge all the buildup. Applying some protein treatment to the hair and scalp will also help in strengthening the hair after the extensions were removed.

Applying scalp treatment products can also help relax the scalp. An example is a scalp treatment product that contains relaxing and calming essential oils such as peppermint. Antiseptic essential oils such as eucalyptus can also help relieve scalp discomforts such as odor and itching. These essential oil blends may help relieve feelings of tightness leftover from the pulling sensation while wearing the hair extensions.

Repair hair after extensions

After hair extensions are removed, there may be instances when you need to do some repair for your own natural hair. Sure, you used hair extensions to look good while your own hair grows naturally to the desired length. However, there may still be a little damage due to the strain of the hair extension weight on the hair roots.

Once the hair extensions were removed, your natural hair will likely be tired, stressed and damaged. There might be some split ends. Your natural hair may also look lackluster and dry. The roots are also likely to be weak.

Do not despair. You have achieved your goal of protecting your growing hair with the hair extensions. Now it's time for you to repair and restore the health of your new hair.

» Use professional products to prevent damage

You should have started applying protective hair care products on your hair before the first strands of the hair extension were installed.

Protected natural hair and proper installation of hair extensions will have minimal damage to your new hair as it grows.

There will still be some damage despite proper preparation and installation. Some of the damages are unavoidable. These can only be limited. This is why it is equally important to continue using protective professional products on your newly grown hair after extensions were removed.

»Removal should be by a trained, skilled professional

Have a professional remove the hair extensions to further reduce any potential damage to the newly grown hair. This is very important if the hair extensions were installed using a bonding agent. These would have to be dissolved before the extension can be removed safe and easy.

Another good thing when going to the professional stylist for removal is after care. After the extensions are removed, the stylist can immediately check your newly grown hair. He/she can trim off any split ends.

» Nourish the new hair

Perform deep conditioning after the extensions are removed. Apply it on your scalp, massaging it well. Use a comb to bring the conditioner evenly through your natural hair.

Get a warm towel and wrap it around your head. You may also use a shower cap or a plastic cap. Leave the conditioner on to work on your scalp and hair for about an hour before rinsing well.

Dry your hair gently but thoroughly. Do not rub your hair strands in between the towel. Comb your hair with a wide-toothed comb to remove tangles. Leave your hair to naturally air dry.

Other Variables That Impact Protection & Growth Of Natural Hair

Although the selected methods above have been known to protect and grow you natural hair, installation of these methods alone may not be the only answer to reach optimal results.

Tips for Maintaining Your Weave

Your weave will have to be properly maintained in order to protect your natural hair underneath as it regrows. Maintenance is also crucial to make your weave look as natural as possible for as long as you need to wear it.

The most important things you need to do for proper maintenance regimen while wearing a weave are the following:

Comb and detangle

The number 1 thing you must remember is to never to comb your hair in the usual manner. You will be ripping through the weave and making a huge mess. Yanking through the weave will damage both the hair extensions and the natural hair growing underneath. Tugging at it will cause your hair to fall.

Comb gently and do not start right at the rots of your natural hair. Start combing and detangling at the bottom or ends of the hair extensions. Work your way up. It is recommended to comb and detangle while the hair is still wet. Weaves can become terribly tangled if not regularly maintained.

Wash

Like all other weaves and your own hair, you need to regularly wash. Regular, in this case, means every 7 to 14 days. If you sweat a lot, you wash your hair and the weave every 7 days.

When washing, make sure to wash the weave and underneath it too. A bottle with an attached nozzle can really help in applying shampoo to your hair underneath the weave.

Mix water and sulfate-free shampoo in the bottle. Apply it to all the crevices and spaces between the braids.

Use your fingertips and lightly massage the scalp, especially in between the braids. Rinse well then apply the shampoo mixture again. Do this at least twice.

When shampooing, start with the scalp and working your way down to the weave. Never ball up your extensions as you would when you shampoo your natural hair. This is a very bad idea. Work your fingers from your scalp down to the hair until you reach the ends.

When you rinse, water will bring the shampoo down through the hair and washing off dirt and oils. Keep your hair extension straight at all times to keep it from tangling and matting.

Always remember to condition. Apply

conditioner with a nozzle to get to the roots of your hair. This is important to nourish your natural hair as it grows underneath your weave. After applying the conditioner, cover your head with a shower cap. Leave the conditioner on for 20 minutes before rinsing.

Dry properly

This is as important as washing your hair and your weave regularly. Make sure that you dry your hair extensions and the braid underneath completely. If not, a really bad smell will develop. Other than that, you will be at huge risk of harboring mildew growth. Moist, dark places like your braid underneath the weave are perfect places for mildew growth. This can be very problematic as various sorts of problems can develop, such as serious scalp infections.

Deal with itchiness

Your scalp will feel very itchy. This can be from the scalp irritation as a result of pulling. The infrequent washing also contributes to the itching.

Never scratch using your fingernails. Never use anything pointed, too such as the tip of a rat-toothed comb. These can scratch your scalp and scabs can form. This can exacerbate itching. The scratches may also get infected.

You can use products meant to soothe itchy scalp. These products were designed to relieve itchiness without disrupting the braids.

Remove properly

The weave will have to be removed by a professional. It will be difficult to prevent damage if you remove it yourself. The weave will have to be removed 6 to 8 weeks after installation.

This is important to allow your natural hair and your scalp to breathe and relax. The constant pull of the braids and the weave on your hair roots may do more harm than help you grow out your natural hair.

If you wait longer, your weave will likely start to look worn out. It will start to look ragged and unhealthy. Your hair underneath will also to mat and may even start falling off.

Before you have your weave removed, it is best to look for signs that it is time. The 3 main signs are:

Braid is loose

The weave is still in its proper place if it is secured well against your scalp via the braid. If the weave is hanging loosely from the braid, it's time for removal.

If you do not remove the weave at this point, your natural hair will be prone to breakage. Loosely hanging weave is pulling on your own real hair too much. Your natural hair is no longer able to support the weight of the weave. If left long enough, hair will break off at the point where the weave is attached.

Blending becomes difficult

Check your crown. If a gap becomes noticeable between your braid and the wefts, it means that your natural hair has significantly grown out. Your tracks are now becoming more visible and it becomes difficult to blend your wefts to your natural hair.

It's time to remove the weave at this point.

Popped thread

Regularly check the thread by running your fingertips along the seam. A popped thread means that the weave has already run its course. This means that the thread can no longer adequately attach the weave to your head. If this happens before the expected course of the weave, just go to the hairstylist. Have your installation checked and reassessed. If you are still a candidate for a weave, then you can always have it reinstalled.

Once the weave shows signs it's time for removal, follow these steps. Remember, the best way is to have a professional remove the weave for you. His/her view is much better than yours. His/her stance (standing behind, beside you) is also more comfortable and allows for greater mobility while removing the weave.

1. Check that the tracks are ready to be removed. One signs is when the braid can be lifted away from your scalp. If the braid cannot be lifted yet, there is a high chance that a good amount of your natural hair will be cut off while the weave is being removed. If the braid can be lifted, weave removal will be much easier and less risky for your natural hair.

2. The weave is pulled up and gathered into a ponytail. Secure it at the top of your head. This will make it easier to work from the bottom of your head upwards. If the weave is short, raise the weave and secure it around your head with clips.

3. Look for the thread used for the weave. Gently and carefully run your fingers along the seam or braid ridge where the hair extension has been sewn in. Isolate the end of the thread and cut it. Use a pair of manicure scissors or needle nose scissors for this. Be careful in cutting because you might cut a large chunk of

your own hair. It may be a better idea to have someone else do this for you if you are having trouble.

You (or the hair stylist) might still cut a bit of you natural hair. Some of the hair that has grown around the seam may be snipped just a little when cutting the thread.

Cut using the tip of the scissors. This will help you to avoid cutting a large amount of your own hair.

At times, if there is a lot of hair growing around the seam, it may be necessary to clip a few of your own real hair. The new hair growth may have grown over the seam, hiding the thread. Clip away a few of your own hair so you can expose the thread.

4. Unweave the thread.

Once cut, start unraveling the thread away from the scalp. You should use both of your hands to pull the extension gently away from the scalp.

Hold your own real hair with one hand, securing the roots to the scalp. This will keep your real hair from getting damaged or breaking while you pull the extension away.

With the other hand, hold the free end of the thread firmly. Tug it lightly in the opposite direction. Keep pulling at the thread lightly to unravel it.

Loosen the seam by wriggling your fingernails in between the braids. You may also use a thin, flat object for this.

You may also need to cut another section in case tangles are formed around the seam. This may be the case if your newly grown hair grew around the seam.

1. Dissolve the thread

Some threads come with a special coating that can be dissolved by special salon hair products. These products make it easier to remove the threads without damaging the hair. These are usually sprayed on the thread and left on for a few minutes.

Get a wide-toothed comb. Run it through your hair, starting from the base of the head towards the top. This will remove any debris in the hair.

2. Find threads and remove

Pull out small sections of hair through the ponytail and remove the threads from within that section. Patiently work through the sections to avoid missing out on weave or thread pieces that might be hidden by your newly grown hair.

It is better to work patiently than having to deal with a chunk of hair later on hanging by its thread.

3. Comb your new hair

Comb your hair with a wide-toothed comb after the hair extensions are removed. This will remove all debris, bonds, threads and pieces of hair extension. Start combing from the top of your head down to the base, at your nape. Then comb from one side to the other and vice versa.

In case there are tangles difficult to remove, try spraying a detangling solution. Do not be hard on tangles as this may cause damage or even cause the hair to break and fall off.

4. Clean your new hair

Use a clarifying shampoo to wash your hair. This will promote a good, relaxing environment for your hair to relax and recover from the stress of having hair extensions.

Bring back nutrients to your hair to promote stronger hair growths. Deeply condition your hair and your scalp.

Diet

Hair nourishment comes from both the products you directly apply to your hair and from what you eat. If you are dehydrated, your hair becomes weak, dull and brittle. If you are well hydrated, you have shinier, smoother and stronger hair. If you eat a balanced meal with all the right vitamins and nutrients, your hair will grow normally and be strong against damage.

A right diet is very important to protect and promote healthy hair growth. This goes for both while wearing a hair extension and after it is removed.

To boost hair nutrition, check that you are eating these foods every day:

Oats

These are excellent sources for proteins,, vitamins and minerals that boost hair growth. Examples include iron, vitamin B, copper, zinc and potassium.

Omega-3s

These can help reduce inflammation resulting from several factors, such as the strain of the extensions. Inflammation can hinder the hair follicles from putting forth healthy hair strands. This can also promote faster hair loss. Reduce inflammation and hair growth proceeds normally, producing healthy, strong hair.

Sweet potatoes

These are rich in beta carotene. The body converts this into vitamin A. In turn, vitamin A is used for the normal production and control of the healthy oils on your scalp.

Beans

These are full of iron, biotin, protein, and zinc that all support healthy, robust hair growth. These can also help in strengthening the hair against breakage.

Poultry

These are healthy sources of proteins that your body can use to grow hair. Proteins are also important in strengthening the hair and protecting it against dryness and breakage.

MATERIALS BEST SUITED FOR YOUR NATURAL HAIR

After the weave is removed, be very careful in how you handle your natural hair. It will be very prone to damage. Choose the products you will use on your natural hair very carefully. Hair products can help strengthen your natural hair and damage it further.

Here are a few of the most important materials you should use on your natural hair.

Dry shampoo

This is one of the must-haves for proper hair maintenance. This is applied on the hair in between regular shampooing.

Applying dry shampoo can help remove the oil and dirt without placing any strain on the hair. Your new hair is likely to be tired, weak and easily damaged. Using regular shampoo and water can be too heavy for your new hair. Use a dry shampoo instead, especially for the first few days. This also avoids oil buildup on the scalp and the hair.

A good product is a keratin-infused dry shampoo. Keratin is an important hair protein. It helps speed up hair growth cycle to promote faster hair regrowth and improve hair loss. This can also boost the rate of hair growth, giving you the length you want within a shorter time span.

Dry shampoo should be free of parabens, sulfate, chlorides and other fillers. These compounds can damage the color of your hair (especially if it is color-treated) and the color of the extensions.

Your dry shampoo should also be talc-free. This will prevent your hair from having visible white residue, which can be very noticeable on darker-colored hair.

Shine & Heat Treatment Spray

Care for real hair against heat damage is important, especially for your new hair growth. There are a number of heat treatment sprays that can protect the hair from getting damaged. This product is applied on the hair before heat-styling, even before blow drying. This will lock in the hair cuticle and make the strands less vulnerable to damage.

Leave-in conditioner

Leave-in conditioners are applied to serve as protection. This conditioner can also help repair any damages before it gets worse.

Leave-in conditioners are also good to use when giving the hair a break from styling. Apply the conditioner on days when you don't heat-style your hair. This can further support repair and rest for your hair.

Remove tangles from your real hair without much pulling force. You can brush continuously from the roots through your hair.

MAINTENANCE FOR NATURAL HAIR AFTER WEAVE IS REMOVED

Expect that your newly grown hair is sensitive after being under the weave for quite some time. This is the tie to be gentle. Once the weight of the weave is off, you have to give your scalp and hair time to relax and recover from all that strain.

Most likely, your new hair has grown all over the place because it was braided. The direction of the strands was not in the natural downward form.

Gently release any tangles by running your fingers gently through your new hair. Loosen the hair then use a wide-toothed comb.

Condition

Apply moisturizing shampoo on your hair to clean it, and then apply conditioner. Comb the hair while there is still conditioner on it. Expect that a few strands will be shed as you comb through your hair. This is normal because of all the normal hair you should have shed while wearing the weave trapped within the braids.

Deep condition

Rinse the conditioner off from your hair. Follow it up with a good deep conditioner. Apply from the scalp to the ends of your hair then wrap with a plastic shower cap. Leave on for about 20 to 30 minutes. Rinse well.

Care for the ends

Next, check the ends of your natural hair. Most likely, there will be a few dead, dry, lightly-colored and rough ends. Trim these off. Clip a tiny length off the ends to promote healthier hair. This can also get rid of all that dryness.

Chapter 7 – Summary

Hair extensions can be worn in many different styles and lengths. It can be installed in various methods. It can serve various purposes.

No matter what your main purpose is in having hair extensions installed and no matter what your choice of method is, one thing is very important to remember- take care of it.

Hair extensions are an investment. It does not matter if the hair extension is inexpensive or very pricey, you have to take care of it.

Maintenance is not just about making sure your hair extensions last long. It is not just about making it look as natural and healthy-looking. It is more about taking care of the hair beneath your own natural hair.

Poorly maintained hair extension will damage your scalp and your hair strands.

Maintenance of Hair Extensions

Proper maintenance of hair extensions will greatly affect the protection rating it will provide for your own natural hair. Even the best hair extensions applied by the most skilled hair stylist will not be able to give the optimum protection if you do not maintain it properly.

Proper maintenance will help make your extensions look great and easy to wear. Proper maintenance will also help make them last longer. Problems and discomforts such as frizzy hair, alopecia and itchy scalp may also be prevented.

The very first thing to know about proper hair extension maintenance is how soon it can be washed. This varies depending on the type of bonds used.

Washing hair is important, just as it is important to shampoo your own hair regularly. Dirt, dust and oils can accumulate. If not regularly removed, these can build up. The buildup can quickly become breeding grounds for bacteria and fungi. These can cause infection that may even worsen hair loss.

Shampoo

Generally, the recommendation is to avoid shampooing the hair for at least 48 hours. This gives the bond time enough to really adhere to the hair. Once settled, the bond will not be easily damaged when it gets wet and exposed to shampoo.

Use only brands that are recommended for use on hair extensions. Most street shampoos (regular shampoos) contain silicone-based ingredients. These can weaken the bonds and speed up break down.

Volumizing shampoos are never recommended for use on hair extensions. This type of shampoo raises the hair cuticles, making the hair look bigger or with greater volume. This effect makes hair more prone to tangling.

Clarifying shampoo can be used on the hair and hair extensions to remove any buildup.

Apply a gentle clarifying shampoo on the hair every 2 to 3 weeks. Removing buildup will allow your regular daily conditioner to set in and work into the hair strands better.

Never wash hair with hot water. This goes when rinsing away shampoo and/or conditioner from your hair.

Extensions should be washed every 2 to 3 days. This will clean the hair regularly enough without getting it dry due to over-shampooing and conditioning.

Conditioning

Special conditioners are available for use on hair extensions that become damaged and dry. Examples are leave-on conditioners/moisturizers, intense hydrator, thermal protectant or cuticle sealer. Apply the product on the hair and leave it on for about 2 minutes. Rinse well.

Deep conditioning is also important. Do this once a week on your hair extensions. Apply the conditioner on the hair extensions. Remember to keep the product away from the bonds. Leave the conditioner on for about 20 to 30 minutes then rinse well. The extra care will give extra boost to your hair extensions' health, look and texture. It may also help improve the lifespan of your hair extensions.

Brushing/Combing

Brush hair regularly to keep it tangle-free. Experts recommend brushing twice a day. Always remember to brush your hair before going to bed.

Use a brush made for hair extensions. Avoid using fine-toothed combs as this can damage the strands and the bonds.

When brushing the hair, start from the scalp and down to the ends of the hair strands. Experts recommend brushing the hair before and after you washed the hair extensions.

Hair products

You can use a few hair products to style your hair extension. Check the labels, especially the ingredients list. Avoid products that have too much oil. Again, grease weighs hair down, both your real hair and your hair extensions. It can also loosen the bonds. Too much oil also traps more dust and dirt along the hair strands.

Avoid products that have too many chemicals in it. These can strip the natural, helpful oils from your hair. These can also destroy the hair cuticle. These can make the hair very dry.

Avoid hair products that contain glycerin, sulfur, silicon and similar compounds. These are harsh on the hair (both real and extension). An example is anti-dandruff shampoo.

Styling

Allow the hair to dry naturally. Avoid applying too much heat, such as blow drying. If you need to use heat such as a flat iron or a blow dryer, use ones that are gentle on the hair. There are heat-styling tools available in gentle ionic configuration. When applying heat, avoid applying it directly on the bonds.

Expert hair stylists suggest using heat protectants on the hair. This will protect the hair extensions from breakage and damage whether you use blow dryer, flat iron, curling iron and other heated styling tools.

Choose the lowest setting when using heated tools for styling. Check that the setting is on low to avoid damage and faster wearing out of the hair extensions.

Conclusion

By now, you should have understood what hair extensions are, the many methods available, and all other pertinent information.

The next step is to assess your hair needs.

Ask yourself these questions:

Do I need hair extensions?

* What type will be easy on my hair? What type can my hair handle? Remember, even the healthiest hair can get damage if the hair extension type is not ideal for the hair type or if the application and maintenance are not done right.

* Do I have what it takes to maintain this type of hair extension? That is, can I go to a salon regularly, once a week or so to get professional care?

Apply the tips and the guides given in this book in planning your next steps.

Your hair is your crowning glory. You need to take care of it to keep it healthy and in top condition always. It does not take expensive salon treatments. A simple regular washing, conditioning and proper de-tangling can turn your locks into the envy of many.

Thank you for reading this book and I hoped you enjoyed it.

For more tips, you can visit my website and social media accounts:

Website: https://www.clishea.co

Pinterest: https://www.pinterest.com/beclishea

Facebook: https://www.facebook.com/beclishea

Instagram: https://www.instagram.com/beclishea